STRONGER THAN SCOLIOSIS

A PARENTS GUIDE TO MAKING THE BEST SCOLIOSIS TREATMENT DECISIONS

Written by the doctors of ScoliSMART

STRONGER THAN
SCOLIOSIS

A PARENTS GUIDE TO MAKING THE BEST SCOLIOSIS TREATMENT DECISIONS

Written by the doctors of ScoliSMART

TABLE OF CONTENT

INTRODUCTION

To the Brave Parents Facing the Challenges of Scoliosis,

When we embark on the journey of parenthood, we expect moments of joy, laughter, and love to fill our days. However, life often throws unexpected challenges our way, and few experiences can be as emotionally taxing as discovering that your child has been diagnosed with scoliosis.

As a parent, you may find yourself caught in a whirlwind of emotions – scared of the unknown, uncertain about the future, frustrated by the lack of control, and confused by the myriad of options presented to you. You're worn out from countless appointments, consultations, and sleepless nights spent worrying. You long for clarity, for someone to guide you through this maze of decisions. You may even find yourself grappling with feelings of guilt, questioning if there was something you could have done differently.

In the midst of this storm, it's natural to feel overwhelmed, to wish for a quick resolution, for this ordeal to be over with. You may find yourself torn between conflicting desires – not knowing exactly what you want, but acutely aware of what you don't want. The thought of bracing or surgery for your child fills you with dread, and you live in fear of making the wrong decision, of inadvertently causing more harm than good.

But amidst all these emotions, I want you to know one thing – you are not alone. There are countless parents out there who have walked this path before you, who have felt the same fears, uncertainties, and frustrations. And it's from their collective wisdom and experiences that this book was born.

Within these pages, you'll find not just information, but empathy and understanding. You'll find stories of resilience, of parents who have navigated the ups and downs of scoliosis with courage and grace. You'll find practical advice, from experts in the field, to help you make informed decisions about your child's care. And most importantly, you'll find hope – hope that no matter how daunting the journey may seem, there is light at the end of the tunnel.

So, to all the parents facing the challenges of scoliosis, I commend you for your strength, your love, and your unwavering commitment to your child's well-being. May this book serve as a beacon of support and guidance as you navigate this difficult terrain, and may you emerge from it stronger, wiser, and more resilient than ever before.

CHAPTER 1:

Understanding the Cause and Impact of Scoliosis

Idiopathic scoliosis is a multifaceted spinal condition defined by an atypical lateral curvature of the spine, presenting challenges for medical practitioners for over 3,500 years! Despite extensive research, the precise cause of scoliosis remains enigmatic, until recently. The researchers at ScoliSMART have pinpointed several factors that could play a role in its development and advancement. Genetic predisposition emerges as a prominent influencer, indicating a hereditary component in some cases. Additionally, imbalances in neurotransmitters and hormones have been implicated in the pathology of idiopathic scoliosis.

Furthermore, environmental factors such as postural habits, muscle imbalances, and asymmetric growth patterns during adolescence are also believed to contribute to the progression of this condition. Understanding these diverse elements that may impact idiopathic scoliosis can aid in developing comprehensive treatment approaches tailored specifically for YOUR CHILD. Early detection and intervention are key in managing scoliosis effectively and preventing potential complications associated with spinal deformities, but children with moderate and severe scoliosis curvatures can and do greatly benefit from these innovative advances in treatment as well.

Scoliosis is a condition that manifests differently in each child, with the severity of the spinal curvature playing a significant role in determining its effects. Mild cases may not cause much discomfort or hinder daily activities, while those with more pronounced curves may experience intense pain, limited mobility, and potential complications that can impact the functionality of vital organs. Therefore, it is crucial to have a thorough comprehension of the causes and consequences of scoliosis to ensure effective treatment and management of this condition.

In addition to physical symptoms, scoliosis can also have psychological and social implications for your child. Dealing with a visible spinal deformity can lead to self-consciousness, low self-esteem, and challenges in social interactions. It is essential for parents to address not only the physical aspects of scoliosis, but also provide support for the mental and emotional well-being of their children.

Traditional treatment options for adolescent idiopathic scoliosis vary depending on factors such as the individual's age, the degree of curvature, and any associated symptoms. In mild cases, monitoring the condition through regular check-ups may recommended, but wastes a golden opportunity for early stage scoliosis intervention while the curve is most flexible and before the conditions gets momentum. Patients with proven curve progression (worsening) are considered more severe cases and may be recommended for bracing or surgical intervention by an orthopedic doctor. Scoliosis bracing is a treatment method that "hopes" to prevent further curvature of the spine, especially in children and adolescents with scoliosis. While bracing has been a longstanding approach in managing scoliosis, the effectiveness of this treatment option remains a topic of debate within the medical community due to inconsistent research data. This lack of consistency raises concerns about relying on bracing for such a crucial aspect of a child's health.

Apart from the uncertain effectiveness, it's essential to consider the significant physical, emotional, and social challenges that prolonged bracing can impose on a child. Long-term adherence to bracing protocols can be demanding and may impact a child's quality of life. Research indicates that only a small percentage, around 10% of children, can tolerate the recommended bracing program effectively.

Given these factors, it's crucial for parents and healthcare providers to weigh the potential benefits against the challenges associated with scoliosis bracing. Alternative treatment options and holistic approaches should also be explored to ensure comprehensive care for children dealing with scoliosis. Regular monitoring by healthcare professionals and open communication with the child about their experience with bracing are key aspects to consider when evaluating the suitability of this treatment method.

Severe spinal curves, typically classified as 50 degrees or more, are often referred for scoliosis surgery to prevent further progression of the condition. The most prevalent surgical procedure for scoliosis is multiple level spinal fusion surgery, where vertebrae are fused together to correct the curvature. However, advancements in medical technology have introduced scoliosis tethering surgeries as an alternative to fusion procedures. These surgeries, known as vertebral body tethering (VBT) or Anterior Scoliosis Correction (ASC), offer a non-fusion option for patients with scoliosis.

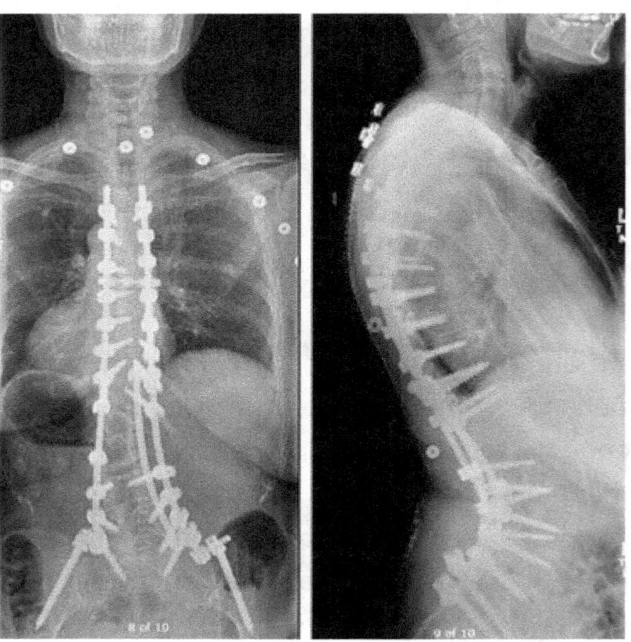

Scoliosis Fusion Surgery, known as
Posterior Pedicle Screw Instrumentation

Scoliosis tethering surgeries involve attaching anchors and flexible cord implants to the spine to guide its growth and correct the curvature gradually over time. Unlike fusion surgery, tethering preserves some spinal flexibility and allows for continued growth in younger patients. This innovative approach to treating scoliosis is particularly beneficial for adolescents and young adults seeking a less invasive surgical solution with potentially better long-term outcomes.

Parents contemplating scoliosis surgery have the right to know that the primary reason for this procedure is to enhance the cosmetic appearance of the spinal deformity and to halt the progression of the curve reliably. It is important to note that scoliosis surgery is not deemed medically necessary and will not have a significant impact on your child's heart or lungs, unless the curvature exceeds 80-90 degrees, which is uncommon even in cases where patients do not undergo treatment. Furthermore, it is crucial to understand that scoliosis surgery does not cure the condition entirely, as scoliosis involves more than just the spine. The surgery replaces a crooked spine, which may be functional and relatively pain-free, with a straighter, but dysfunctional fused or tethered spine that could be susceptible to chronic pain. It is essential for parents to weigh the potential benefits and risks associated with scoliosis surgery carefully before making a decision for their child's treatment, because it is permanent and can not be reversed.

Scoliosis-specific exercises are designed to target and strengthen the muscles that support the spine, offering a key strategy in managing scoliosis and enhancing long-term posture memory for patients. By engaging in these exercises, kids with scoliosis can train their brains to naturally maintain a less twisted and crooked spinal position. This muscle strengthening not only helps in improving posture, but also aids in reducing pain and discomfort associated with scoliosis. Consistent practice of these specialized exercises can lead to increased flexibility, better spinal alignment, and enhanced overall quality of life for scoliosis patients. It is important for individuals with scoliosis to work closely with a ScoliSMART doctor to develop a personalized exercise routine that suits their specific condition and goals.

Educating patients and their families about scoliosis, its potential effects, and available treatment options is essential for empowering them to make informed decisions about their care. By taking a holistic and truly comprehensive approach that addresses both the physical spinal curve and genetic, neurotransmitter, and hormonal aspects of the WHOLE scoliosis condition, we can now support your child in a way never before thought possible.

CHAPTER 2:

Genetic Factors and Other Problems Associated With Scoliosis

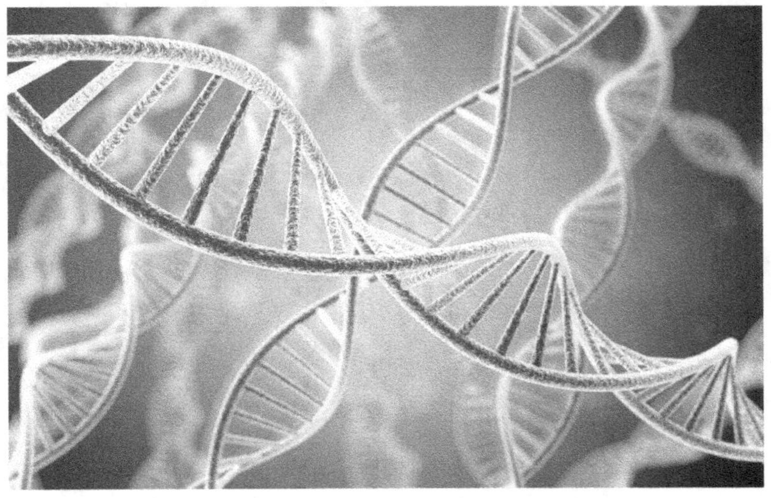

While genetics play a significant role in the development of idiopathic scoliosis, most doctors and researchers consider the exact cause of this condition remains unknown. However, our studies have revealed a strong correlation between specific genetic markers and the likelihood of developing scoliosis. However, it is crucial to note that about 22% of individuals with these genetic markers will not develop the condition. Other factors such as neurotransmitter imbalances, hormonal changes, and environmental influences also contribute to the onset of and progression of idiopathic scoliosis. Further research is needed to unravel the complex interplay between genetics and other physiological factors in the manifestation of this disorder.

Our research has identified 28 specific genetic variants that are associated with idiopathic scoliosis, shedding light on the underlying genetic factors contributing to the development of this condition. These genetic variants play a role in the regulation of bone growth, digestive function, neurotransmitter patterns, hormone metabolism, and ultimately, spinal alignment. Understanding the genetic basis of idiopathic scoliosis is crucial for early detection, personalized treatment approaches, and advancing research efforts aimed at improving patient outcomes.

Kids with a family history of idiopathic scoliosis may have an increased risk of developing the condition due to these genetic factors. Genetic testing and screening for these specific variants can help identify individuals at higher risk and enable proactive management strategies to prevent or mitigate the progression of scoliosis. By unraveling the genetic complexities associated with idiopathic scoliosis, researchers and healthcare providers can enhance diagnostic accuracy, develop targeted therapies, and ultimately improve the quality of life for kids affected by this condition.

DNA testing for scoliosis can provide valuable insights into the genetic factors associated with idiopathic scoliosis in your child. By analyzing your child's DNA, our doctors can identify specific genetic markers or variations that may predispose them to developing this condition. This information can be crucial in understanding the underlying causes of scoliosis and determining the most effective treatment and management strategies for your child.

Moreover, DNA testing can help predict the progression of scoliosis, allowing for early intervention and personalized care plans. By identifying genetic risk factors early on, we can implement targeted scoliosis supplement interventions to potentially prevent or minimize the severity of spinal curvature in children with a higher genetic predisposition to scoliosis.

In addition to aiding in diagnosis and treatment planning, DNA testing for scoliosis can also offer valuable information for families regarding the hereditary nature of the condition. Understanding the genetic basis of idiopathic scoliosis can empower parents to make informed decisions about their child's healthcare and take proactive steps to monitor their spinal health.

Overall, incorporating DNA testing into the evaluation and management of scoliosis can significantly enhance clinical outcomes by enabling personalized care based on individual genetic profiles. It represents a promising avenue for advancing precision medicine approaches and improving long-term outcomes for children affected by idiopathic scoliosis.

Neurotransmitter imbalances also play a significant role in the development and progression of idiopathic scoliosis. Studies have suggested a correlation between neurotransmitter imbalances and the onset of scoliosis, as well as associated issues commonly observed in children with the condition, such as depression, sleep disturbances, anxiety, and attention-deficit/hyperactivity disorder (ADHD).

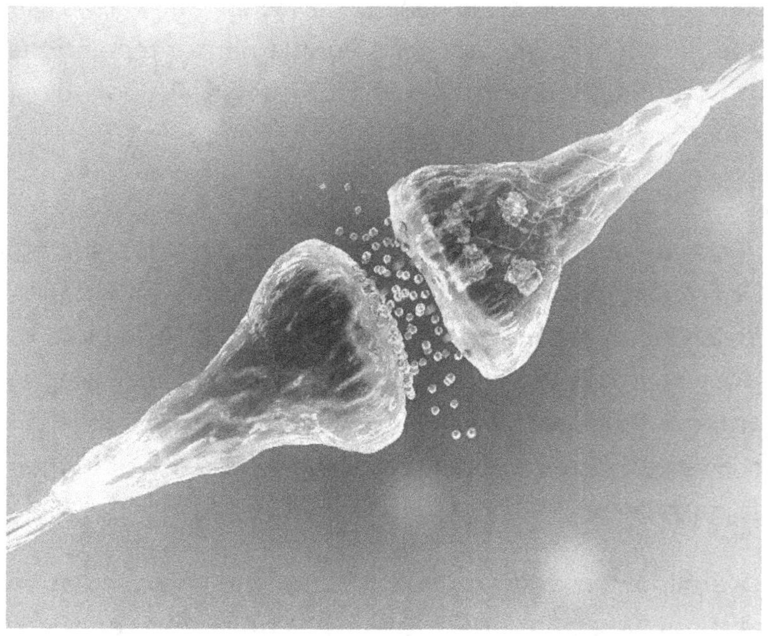

A microscopic view of a neuron end terminal. The small dots are neurotransmitters such as serotonin that are responsible for allowing nerve impulses to cross the gap over to the next neuron.

Serotonin, a neurotransmitter responsible for regulating mood and emotions, has been particularly implicated in scoliosis. Low levels of serotonin have been linked to depressive symptoms often seen in children with scoliosis. Similarly, imbalances in dopamine and norepinephrine levels may contribute to anxiety and ADHD symptoms in these kids as well.

Understanding the role of neurotransmitters in scoliosis can open avenues for potential treatment strategies that target not only the physical aspects of the condition, but also address the associated mental health challenges. Further research into this area could lead to more holistic approaches to managing idiopathic scoliosis and improving the overall well-being of patients affected by this condition.

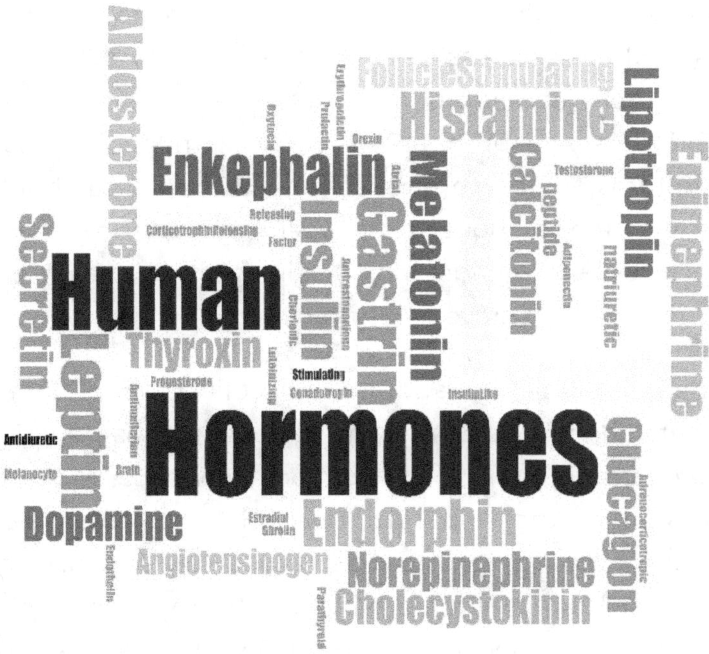

Hormones are the main signaling chemicals in the body. Without them, nothing works correctly.

Hormone levels and their balance, particularly between estrogen and progesterone, have been identified as factors that can impact the progression of scoliosis curves. Research suggests that these hormones play a role in the development and worsening of scoliosis, especially during periods of rapid growth such as puberty. Estrogen, for instance, has been associated with an increased risk of scoliosis progression, potentially due to its effects on bone density and growth plates. Progesterone, on the other hand, may have a protective effect against scoliosis advancement.

Understanding the influence of hormone levels on scoliosis can be crucial in managing the condition, especially in cases where progression needs to be monitored closely. Hormonal fluctuations during different life stages or conditions like pregnancy can also impact scoliosis symptoms and curve progression. Further research into the intricate relationship between hormone levels and scoliosis may provide valuable insights for treatment approaches and preventive measures.

When it comes to addressing scoliosis in children, understanding the underlying factors such as genetics, neurotransmitter levels, and hormone imbalances is crucial. By targeting these specific issues with tailored scoliosis supplementation, it is possible to not only enhance the effectiveness of treatment protocols, but to also minimize the risk of the spinal curvature worsening as the child develops. Moreover, addressing these factors can lead to overall improvements in the child's health and well-being.

It is essential to work closely with ScoliSMART specialists to determine the most suitable supplementation approach for each child based on their individual needs and circumstances. By taking a comprehensive and targeted approach to scoliosis management, parents can help support their child's health and development effectively.

CHAPTER 3:

The Importance of Early Stage Intervention and Getting Ahead of Scoliosis

While it is commonly understood that younger children with smaller spinal curves tend to respond more favorably to treatment compared to older children with more severe scoliosis curves, there is still hope for improvement even in cases of larger curves. Early intervention and monitoring are crucial in managing scoliosis, as it allows for the implementation of appropriate treatments such as Small Curve Camp and genetic testing to help prevent further curvature progression.

In cases where scoliosis has progressed significantly, additional options may be considered to treat the spinal curve and alleviate associated symptoms. These options may include more extensive testing, the ScoliSMART Activity Suit, or even extended Scoliosis BootCamp programs for severe cases. It's important for kids with scoliosis, regardless of age or curve size, to work closely with a ScoliSMART doctor to develop a personalized treatment plan that addresses their specific needs and improves their quality of life.

Regular monitoring and adherence to treatment recommendations can help minimize the impact of scoliosis on daily activities and overall well-being. It's essential for parents and caregivers to support children with scoliosis throughout their treatment journey and encourage them to stay positive and proactive in managing their condition. By taking proactive steps and seeking appropriate care, children living with scoliosis can lead fulfilling lives and maintain good spinal health.

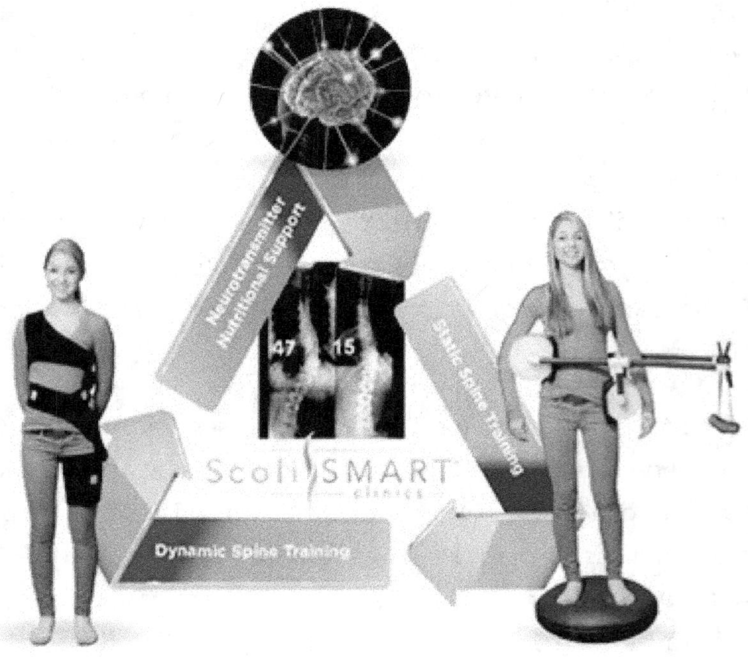

ScoliSMART is the only treatment system currently available that evaluates so many different components of scoliosis to encourage lasting spine change.

ScoliSMART's pioneering non-bracing and non-surgical methodology for addressing moderate to severe scoliosis marks a significant departure from traditional approaches. This progressive treatment approach surpasses mere symptom alleviation by delving into the underlying factors contributing to scoliosis. Through a comprehensive program encompassing specific exercises, tailored therapies, and nutritional assistance, ScoliSMART intends not only to arrest the progression of scoliosis, but also to improve spinal alignment and overall functionality.

The focus on identifying muscle imbalances and neurological issues sets ScoliSMART apart as it seeks to address the root causes of scoliosis rather than merely treating its symptoms. By adopting a comprehensive approach that targets the core issues associated with scoliosis, ScoliSMART offers patients the potential for improved outcomes and long-term spinal health.

The ScoliSMART methodology stands out for its ability to address scoliosis symptoms effectively, offering patients relief without the discomfort and limitations often associated with bracing or surgery. This approach appeals to individuals seeking a holistic and personalized treatment plan tailored to their specific requirements. ScoliSMART's customized plans are designed to comprehensively manage every aspect of the condition, ensuring that patients receive targeted care that caters to their unique needs. By focusing on individualized treatment strategies, ScoliSMART aims to provide a more comfortable and effective alternative for those dealing with scoliosis.

In addition to its personalized approach, ScoliSMART stands out for its integration of diverse therapeutic modalities and emphasis on individualized care, presenting a complete solution for managing scoliosis. By prioritizing sustainable outcomes and an improved quality of life, ScoliSMART underscores its commitment to providing an advanced and tailored approach for individuals looking for a proactive strategy to address their scoliosis condition.

Furthermore, the patient-centric ethos of ScoliSMART emphasizes the importance of offering individualized care that considers each patient's specific needs and preferences. This approach not only differentiates ScoliSMART from traditional treatment methods, but also highlights its dedication to empowering patients in their journey towards managing scoliosis effectively and enhancing their overall well-being.

CHAPTER 4:

Benefits of Scoliosis Exercises in Managing the Condition

Treating your child's scoliosis condition with an exercise and rehabilitation program offers numerous advantages. Firstly, it is a non-invasive approach that can help improve your child's spinal curvature without the need for surgery. By engaging in exercises tailored to their condition, your child becomes actively involved in their treatment, empowering them to take charge of their health. Additionally, such programs often incorporate the latest treatment methodologies and techniques backed by research and studies, ensuring that your child receives the most effective care available. Regular physical activity can also strengthen muscles around the spine, improve posture, and potentially reduce pain associated with scoliosis. Moreover, an exercise and rehabilitation program can promote overall physical well-being and enhance flexibility and mobility in children with scoliosis. It is important to consult with a ScoliSMART doctor who specializes in scoliosis treatment to design a personalized exercise plan suitable for your child's needs and condition.

Non-invasive scoliosis treatment should always be the first approach when managing this condition. Non-invasive treatments focus on correcting spinal curvature and preventing further progression of scoliosis, without the need for surgery. These treatments may include reflexive response training, chiropractic care, and specific exercises targeted at strengthening core muscles and improving posture.

In addition to these treatments, specific exercises such as stretching, strengthening, and postural exercises can help manage scoliosis symptoms. These exercises are tailored to each individual's curve pattern and severity to optimize results.

Choosing non-invasive treatments as the primary approach not only avoids the risks associated with surgery, but also promotes overall spinal health and function. Regular monitoring by your ScoliSMART doctor is essential to track progress and make adjustments to the treatment plan as needed. By prioritizing non-invasive methods, kids with scoliosis (and their parents) can effectively manage their condition and maintain a good quality of life.

Active involvement of a child in their treatment not only enhances muscle strength, but also helps in re-coordinating muscle firing patterns. This active participation creates essential feedback loops from the muscles to the brain, aiding in the development of a new and improved "posture memory". By engaging in these exercise therapy sessions that require little physical effort and concentration, children can effectively retrain their muscles and reinforce proper posture habits. This process is crucial for long-term postural correction and overall musculoskeletal health. Encouraging children to take ownership of their treatment can have far-reaching benefits, extending beyond just their immediate health concerns. When children are actively involved in managing their own health, they develop a sense of responsibility and empowerment. This not only leads to better outcomes in terms of adherence to treatment plans, but also fosters a deeper understanding of their body mechanics. By being more aware of how their bodies function and respond to different treatments, children can make informed decisions about their health as they grow older.

Also, instilling a sense of ownership in children promotes the development of healthier habits from a young age. When children understand the importance of taking care of their bodies and actively participate in their treatment, they are more likely to adopt positive behaviors that support their overall well-being. These habits can have long-term effects on their health outcomes and quality of life.

By encouraging children to be proactive about their health and treatment, parents empower them to become advocates for their own well-being. This not only benefits the child in the present, but also equips them with valuable skills and attitudes that will serve them throughout their lives.

Rehabilitation and exercise programs play a crucial role in the comprehensive treatment of scoliosis, a condition characterized by an abnormal sideways curvature of the spine, but also linked to genetic, neurotransmitter, and hormone issues. These programs are designed based on the latest research and understanding of scoliosis to effectively manage symptoms and improve quality of life for individuals with this spinal deformity.

Physical therapy exercises are tailored to strengthen the muscles surrounding the spine, promote flexibility, and correct spinal alignment. These exercises not only help alleviate pain and discomfort associated with scoliosis, but also prevent further progression of the spinal curvature. By targeting specific muscle groups, children can enhance their core stability and overall spinal health.

Our rehabilitation programs for scoliosis often incorporate various techniques such as Torso Trainer exercises used during Scoliosis BootCamp. Pilates, Schroth, yoga, and aquatic therapy cannot and do not provide the "reflexive response" type reaction necessary to target the part of the brain that controls spinal alignment. These specialized approaches claim to address individual needs and target specific areas of weakness or imbalance in the spine, but fail to create a new posture memory.

It is important for parents and their children with scoliosis to work closely with ScoliSMART doctors who are scoliosis exercise specialists, to develop a personalized rehabilitation plan that suits their unique condition and goals. By actively engaging in rehabilitation and exercise programs that align with current treatment options for scoliosis, patients can optimize their outcomes and enhance their overall spinal health and function.

CHAPTER 5:

The ScoliSMART Approach
to Scoliosis Treatment

The ScoliSMART approach is the most comprehensive approach for treating scoliosis ever developed. It includes the only scoliosis DNA testing, scoliosis-specific neurotransmitter and hormone testing with highly targeted supplementation. Intensive Small Curve Camp (mild scoliosis) and Scoliosis BootCamp (moderate to severe scoliosis) in-office programs, and the patented ScoliSMART Activity Suit.

Scoliosis DNA testing, scoliosis-specific neurotransmitter and hormone testing with highly targeted supplementation can provide valuable insights into the underlying factors contributing to scoliosis. By analyzing an individual's DNA, healthcare providers can identify genetic predispositions that may influence the development and progression of scoliosis. Additionally, Neurotransmitter and hormone testing can provide valuable insights into potential imbalances that may be influencing the scoliosis condition. By analyzing levels of neurotransmitters such as serotonin, dopamine, and histamine, as well as hormones like progesterone and estrogen, ScoliSMART doctors can better understand the underlying physiological factors contributing to the development or progression of the curve.

Imbalances in neurotransmitters can affect muscle function and coordination, which are crucial for maintaining proper spinal alignment. Hormonal fluctuations, especially during growth periods or due to conditions like hormonal disorders, can also impact bone density and growth patterns, potentially exacerbating spinal curvature associated with scoliosis.

Identifying these imbalances through testing allows for more targeted treatment approaches that address not only the structural aspects of scoliosis but also the biochemical factors that may be influencing its course. By integrating this total understanding of the body's biochemistry, ScoliSMART can offer more comprehensive care for kids with scoliosis, improving outcomes and quality of life.

With this detailed information, tailored supplementation protocols can be designed to address specific deficiencies or imbalances, potentially supporting spinal health and reducing the symptoms associated with scoliosis. This personalized approach will optimize treatment outcomes for your child in their battle with scoliosis.

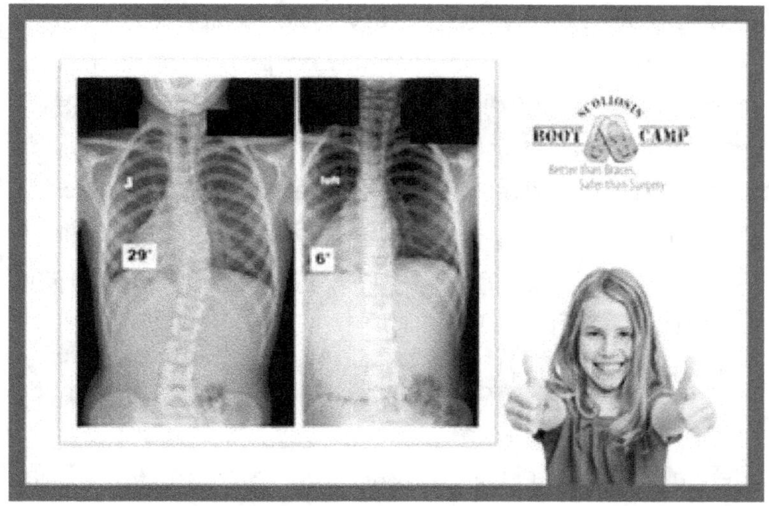

Scoliosis BootCamp is a great way to get a jumpstart on the management process, and to set a foundation for success.

Intensive Small Curve Camp (mild scoliosis) and Scoliosis BootCamp (moderate to severe scoliosis) are specialized, in-office programs designed to address different levels of scoliosis.

The Intensive Small Curve Camp is designed to offer proactive care for kids dealing with mild scoliosis. This program is dedicated to providing personalized treatment plans that may consist of a combination of exercises, stretches, and spinal adjustments customized to the unique curvature of each participant's needs. The primary goal of this program is to intervene in scoliosis during its early stages, with participants striving to halt the advancement of the condition and enhance the alignment of their spine.

In addition to physical interventions, the camp may also incorporate educational components aimed at empowering children with scoliosis by equipping them with knowledge about their condition and ways to manage it effectively. By taking a proactive approach through targeted treatments and lifestyle modifications, participants in the Intensive Small Curve Camp are working towards better spinal health and overall well-being.

The Scoliosis BootCamp is tailored for individuals grappling with moderate to severe scoliosis. This structured program offers a more intensive approach to treatment, which may include the use of the ScoliSMART Activity Suit, specialized exercises, and in some cases, additional testing, based on the extent of the spinal curvature. The primary objective of the Scoliosis BootCamp is to alleviate symptoms, reduce the existing spinal curve, and create spinal stability despite advanced stages of scoliosis.

Participants in the Scoliosis BootCamp can expect a personalized treatment plan that addresses their specific condition. The program may encompass a range of therapeutic modalities designed to strengthen core muscles, improve posture memory, and enhance flexibility. Additionally, participants will receive guidance on proper body mechanics and lifestyle modifications to support their spinal health in the long term.

Furthermore, the Scoliosis BootCamp provides a supportive environment where your child can connect with their doctor, fellow patients, and the expert staff members. This collaborative approach fosters a sense of community and empowerment among participants as they navigate their scoliosis journey. By combining education, exercises, and individualized care, the Scoliosis BootCamp equips your child with the tools they need to effectively manage their condition and strive for better spinal health.

Both programs emphasize the importance of early intervention and customized care to effectively address varying degrees of scoliosis. Participants can benefit from expert guidance, personalized treatment plans, and a supportive environment focused on improving spinal health and functional outcomes.

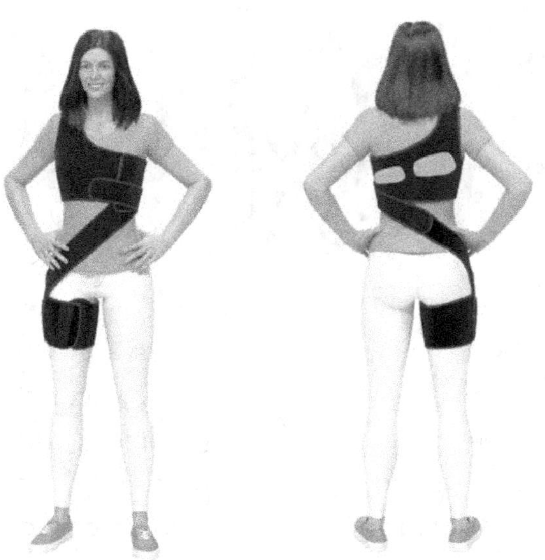

The patented ScoliSMART Activity Suit

The ScoliSMART Activity Suit revolutionizes scoliosis treatment by being the first personalized rehabilitation system for this condition. By harnessing the natural movements of walking and running, the suit automatically works to untwist the scoliosis curve. Not only does it address the curvature of the spine, but it also strengthens muscles, improves muscle coordination, and helps establish a new muscle/posture memory for a more aligned spinal position in the long term.

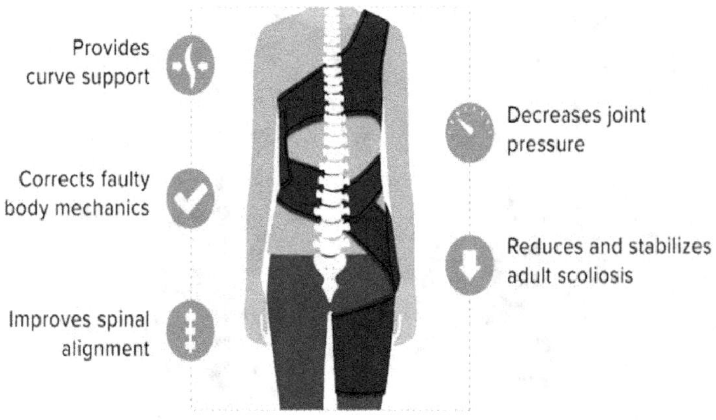

The ScoliSMART Activity Suit presents a groundbreaking method that caters to individuals, particularly children in their developmental stages, grappling with scoliosis. Its non-invasive and proactive nature sets it apart from conventional treatments such as braces or surgical interventions. This innovative approach integrates daily activities into the treatment regimen, offering a comfortable and efficient way to address scoliosis.

Central to the ScoliSMART Activity Suit is its emphasis on improving muscle functionality and encouraging proper spinal alignment. By personalizing the rehabilitation process, this system not only manages scoliosis, but also instills optimism in those navigating this condition. Through its holistic approach that prioritizes enhancing muscle strength and promoting spinal health, the ScoliSMART Activity Suit represents a beacon of hope for parents and their children seeking alternatives to traditional scoliosis treatments.

CHAPTER 6:

How the ScoliSMART Approach Differs from Traditional Methods

The ScoliSMART treatment approach is a comprehensive method that sets itself apart by not only addressing the outward symptom of scoliosis, which is the curvature of the spine, but also concentrating on treating the fundamental causes of the condition. In contrast to conventional treatments such as back braces and spinal surgeries, which primarily focus on correcting the spinal curve, ScoliSMART takes a comprehensive approach towards all facets of scoliosis. By targeting the underlying issues of the condition, this innovative approach strives to offer lasting advantages and mitigate potential complications that could emerge if left unattended.

Furthermore, ScoliSMART incorporates advanced technologies and personalized treatment plans tailored to each individual's unique condition. These customized protocols can include exercises, nutritional guidance, and other non-invasive methods aimed at not just managing scoliosis, but also improving overall spinal health and functionality. By emphasizing early detection and proactive intervention, ScoliSMART advocates for a proactive stance in managing scoliosis to enhance patients' quality of life and prevent progression to more severe stages of the condition.

While back braces and surgeries can offer temporary solutions by only addressing the curvature of the spine in scoliosis patients, they may not always target all the root causes of the condition. It's essential to understand that scoliosis is a complex condition that involves more than just the physical alignment of the spine. Factors such as muscle imbalances, postural habits, and even emotional stress can play a role in the progression of scoliosis. In addition to using back braces and surgery for a temporary solution to the much bigger problem, some parents also hope incorporating holistic approaches like general physical therapy, chiropractic care, and regular exercises to strengthen core muscles and improve posture hoping they can be beneficial. Unfortunately, these non-invasive methods also fail to focus on addressing the underlying issues contributing to scoliosis, and are just correcting spinal alignment temporarily.

Adopting a comprehensive treatment plan that includes nutritional support, reflexive response techniques, and regular monitoring by your ScoliSMART doctor can help your child manage their condition effectively in the long term. By addressing both the physical and the underlying aspects of scoliosis, your child can experience improved quality of life and better overall health outcomes. Without tackling these root causes, your child will not achieve long-lasting results and could encounter recurring issues down the line. What sets the ScoliSMART treatment approach apart is its comprehensive methodology that takes into account a wide range of scoliosis-related challenges, offering a more holistic solution for patients. In addition to addressing spinal curvature, this approach considers factors such as muscle imbalances, neurological abnormalities, and genetic predispositions that play a role in scoliosis development and progression. By targeting these various components simultaneously, ScoliSMART aims to provide more effective and sustainable outcomes for kids dealing with scoliosis.

ScoliSMART's innovative approach to scoliosis treatment is a comprehensive method that delves deeper than just symptom management. Rather than merely addressing the outward signs of scoliosis, ScoliSMART targets the underlying causes of the condition. This unique strategy concentrates on improving overall spinal health and function, providing patients with a more enduring treatment solution. By proactively correcting imbalances and fortifying supporting structures, ScoliSMART strives to achieve superior results, ultimately enhancing the quality of life for every child dealing with scoliosis.

In addition to focusing on spinal health, ScoliSMART's approach often includes personalized exercises, nutritional guidance, and other natural methods to optimize treatment outcomes. By taking a multifaceted approach that considers various aspects of a patient's well-being, ScoliSMART sets itself apart in the realm of scoliosis treatment. This proactive and individualized methodology reflects a commitment to not only managing scoliosis but also fostering long-term spinal health and overall wellness for patients.

In addition to traditional treatments that often focus on symptom management, ScoliSMART's comprehensive approach considers the underlying factors contributing to scoliosis development. By emphasizing long-term spinal health and function, patients may experience lasting benefits and improved well-being. This comprehensive strategy not only addresses the physical aspects of scoliosis, but also promotes overall health and quality of life for individuals seeking effective and sustainable treatment options.

CHAPTER 7:

Success Stories and Testimonials from ScoliSMART Parents and Patients

The ScoliSMART approach has been a blessing for numerous children and parents in their battle against scoliosis. Over the years, we have had the privilege of working with countless parents and their children who have embraced this approach to combat scoliosis for every degree of curvature. Through dedication and perseverance, these families have found success in managing and improving their condition using the innovative techniques offered by ScoliSMART. The positive impact of this approach on the lives of those affected by scoliosis is truly remarkable, and we are grateful to have played a part in their journey towards better spinal health.

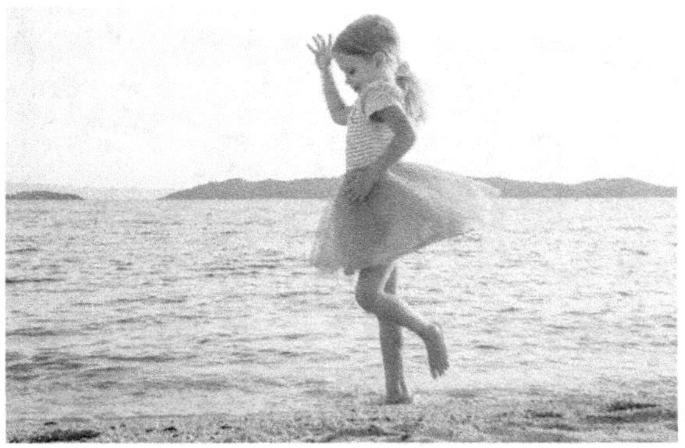

Brittany's proactive scoliosis treatment!

Small Curve Camp is a proactive program that caters to individuals with mild scoliosis, offering a holistic approach to managing and improving their condition. Through a combination of reflexive response exercises, nutritional therapies, and support, the camp has successfully helped her strengthen her core muscles, improved the posture, reduced the curve and created long-term spinal stability.

Participants at Small Curve Camp not only benefit from targeted exercises designed to correct spinal alignment but also receive education on proper body mechanics and ergonomics to prevent further progression of the condition. The camp's comprehensive approach addresses the physical, emotional, and mental aspects of living with scoliosis, empowering individuals to take control of their health and well-being.

Success stories from other kids who have attended Small Curve Camp are a testament to the effectiveness of its specialized programs. Many have reported reduced pain levels, increased flexibility, and a sense of accomplishment after completing the camp. By focusing on individualized care and personalized treatment plans, Small Curve Camp continues to make a positive impact on kids diagnosed with mild scoliosis.

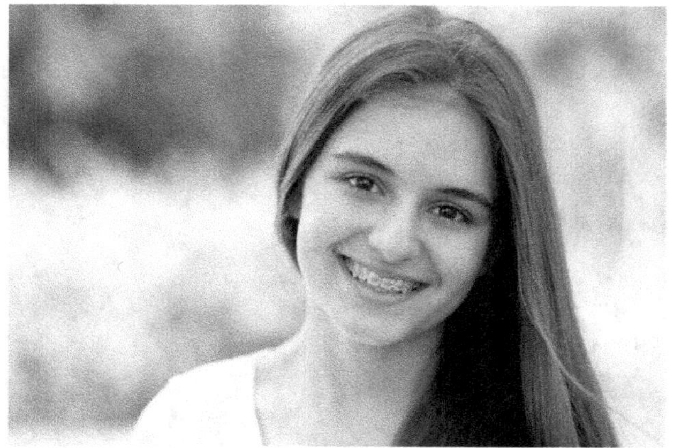

Amy was able to ditch her scoliosis brace!

After completing an intensive 5-day Scoliosis BootCamp program, Amy experienced such significant improvement in her condition that she no longer required her scoliosis brace. The intensive program likely consisted of a combination of targeted exercises, scoliosis supplements based on her test results, and the ScoliSMART Activity Suit to help realign her spine and strengthen the surrounding muscles. Her remarkable outcome showcases the effectiveness of specialized programs like the Scoliosis BootCamp in providing relief and improved quality of life for kids dealing with scoliosis. It also highlights the importance of early intervention and proactive measures in managing spinal conditions.

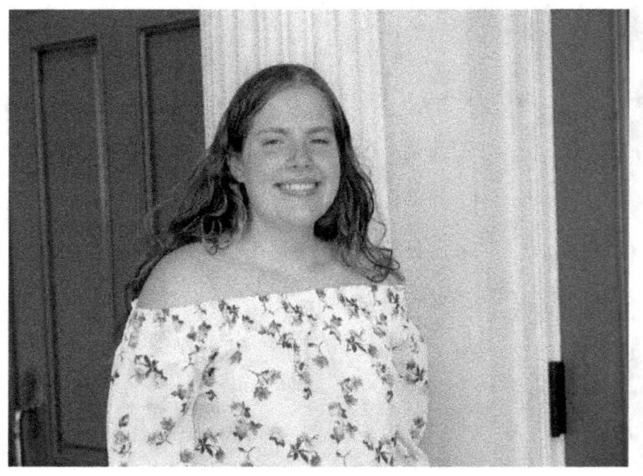

Jennifer skipped the surgery!

While Jennifer may have initially been recommended spinal fusion surgery for her scoliosis, her experience at the 10-day Scoliosis BootCamp proved to be transformative. The intensive program likely involved a combination of nutrient therapies, targeted exercises, stretching treatments, and the ScoliSMART Activity Suit for improving spinal alignment and muscle strength. By actively participating in the BootCamp, Jennifer has successfully avoided the need for invasive surgery by addressing her scoliosis through non-invasive methods. This highlights the potential effectiveness of alternative treatments and rehabilitation programs for managing scoliosis and improving quality of life, without resorting to surgical intervention.

Parents seek the most effective scoliosis treatment for their children while ensuring that their kids can still enjoy a normal childhood. The treatment approach for scoliosis must not only be successful in correcting the spinal curvature but also prioritize maintaining the child's quality of life throughout the treatment journey. It is essential to consider treatments that not only address the physical aspects of scoliosis, but also take into account the emotional well-being and social development of the child. Collaborating with healthcare professionals who specialize in pediatric scoliosis can help parents navigate treatment options that are both medically effective and age-appropriate for their children. Additionally, providing a supportive environment at home and school can contribute to the overall well-being of a child undergoing scoliosis treatment, allowing them to thrive academically, socially, and emotionally despite their condition.

CHAPTER 8:

The Doctors of ScoliSMART

In the realm of scoliosis care, the ScoliSMART group of dedicated chiropractic physicians stand out for their unwavering commitment to treating scoliosis patients exclusively. These doctors have devoted their life's work to advancing the understanding and management of scoliosis, continually contributing to the body of knowledge through published research, innovative technologies, and treatment opportunities. What sets them apart is not only their professional expertise but also their personal connection to scoliosis, as some of them are parents of children with complex medical conditions themselves.

These doctors have made scoliosis their primary focus, dedicating their careers to providing comprehensive care and support for individuals with spinal curvature abnormalities. With a deep understanding of the complexities of scoliosis and a commitment to holistic, patient-centered care, they strive to empower their patients to achieve optimal spinal health and quality of life.

Driven by a passion for advancing the field of scoliosis care, these experts continually contribute to the body of knowledge through rigorous research and scholarly publications. By conducting clinical studies, case reports, and outcome assessments, they seek to enhance our understanding of scoliosis pathogenesis, treatment efficacy, and long-term outcomes.

In addition to their contributions to research, our doctors are at the forefront of innovation, inventing and creating new technologies and treatment opportunities for individuals with scoliosis. From advanced bracing systems and orthotic devices to novel therapeutic approaches and rehabilitation protocols, they strive to push the boundaries of scoliosis care and improve patient outcomes.

Many of our doctors have a deeply personal connection to scoliosis, as they are parents of children who have been diagnosed with the condition. This firsthand experience fuels their passion for scoliosis care and drives their dedication to improving treatment options and outcomes for all individuals affected by spinal curvature abnormalities. As both healthcare providers and parents, they understand the challenges and complexities of navigating the journey with scoliosis and are committed to supporting patients and families every step of the way.

In conclusion, the ScoliSMART specialists who exclusively work with scoliosis patients are true pioneers in the field of spinal health and wellness. Through their dedication, expertise, and compassion, they are transforming the landscape of scoliosis care, advancing research, innovation, and treatment opportunities, and providing hope and healing to individuals and families affected by spinal curvature abnormalities. Their tireless efforts exemplify the profound impact that healthcare providers can have on the lives of those living with scoliosis, inspiring hope, empowerment, and resilience in the face of adversity.

www.ingramcontent.com/pod-product-compliance
Lightning Source LLC
Chambersburg PA
CBHW051708250726

48653CB00007B/2922